OUR DAILY CONNECTION:

A Journal for Brain Illness Caregivers
to Share Facts, Fun and Feelings

Joni James Aldrich

ISBN: 1456477250

ISBN-13: 9781456477257

Printed in the United States of America

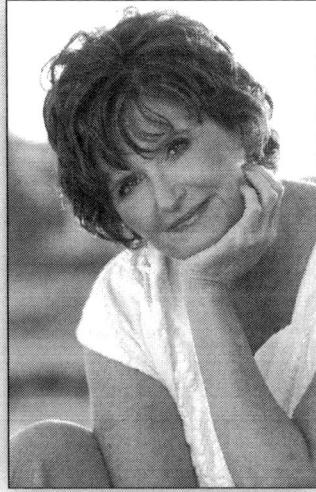

AUTHOR'S PAGE

Joni Aldrich, author and speaker. This is the sixth book that Joni has written on how to survive caregiving, cancer, brain illness, and grief. This journey began after she lost her husband, Gordon, to metastatic brain cancer, a disease with symptoms similar to dementia, Alzheimer's disease and a stroke. She believes that there is an unmet need for practical information to help patients and their families, so she continues to research and write books about the daily rigors of living when a chronic, life-threatening illness invades your world.

Joni believes that she has been prepared throughout her lifetime to write books and reach out to people affected by life's most difficult challenges. Turning her own devastation at the loss of Gordon into hope for others is no easy task, but Joni believes that she is destined to follow this path.

While Joni was completing this manuscript, her mother was under hospice care for lung cancer. They brainstormed with the hospice aide, who also cares for dementia and Alzheimer's disease patients. Some of the contributions throughout this book were from that very special day.

Special thanks to:

Martha James (who passed away on February 24, 2011)

Pam McClendon, hospice aide

INTRODUCTION

The statistics are sobering—now and well into the future—until a cure is found for dementia and Alzheimer's disease. In the United States, approximately four million people have dementia (Alzheimer's disease is a form of dementia), although the number may be as high as five million. If you're wondering why there isn't a more definitive number, it's because brain illnesses (except for tumor detection in brain cancer patients) are difficult to definitively diagnose.

"While there have been significant advances in diagnostic testing methods for Alzheimer's (brain scans and spinal taps may detect certain biomarkers of the disease even in its pre-clinical stage), currently, there is no single test that can diagnose Alzheimer's disease with 100% accuracy. Doctors must use a variety of assessments and laboratory measurements to make what we call a 'differential diagnosis'. They focus on ruling out all other possible causes for the symptoms. A diagnosis is said to be either possible (not all other causes can be ruled out) or probable (all other causes have been ruled out). Presently, a definitive diagnosis of Alzheimer's is possible only by examining brain tissue after death."

~ *From the Fisher Center for Alzheimer's Research Foundation Web site*

There are other types of brain illnesses, such as stroke, malignant and non-malignant brain tumors, and Parkinson's disease. After living through the final days of my husband's life with metastatic brain cancer, I have a healthy respect for caregivers of any brain illness. If the diagnosis is dementia or Alzheimer's disease, you are possibly facing years or decades of caregiving.

Whether you have time to adapt and learn or not, the stress can be truly unbearable at times. I highly recommend reading either ***Connecting through Compassion: Guidance for Family and Friends of a Brain Cancer Patient*** or ***Understanding with Compassion: Help for Loved Ones and Caregivers of a Brain Illness Patient.*** I'm convinced that these books will smooth the rough edges for both the caregiver and care receiver (directly or indirectly). You can continue to love and live after a brain illness diagnosis.

Going forward in your daily walk with a brain illness patient, journaling is an important documentation tool. Kymberly Holland (a friend and widow of a brain cancer patient) explains the importance of journaling this way:

"I started journaling as a daily log to chronicle my husband's seizures, and eventually added what he was doing at the time that might have caused them. That was how I was able to pinpoint when a seizure might happen. Then, I started adding in his feelings after the events—how they correlated with the types of seizures he was having. I showed his doctors the diary, and told them my conclusions of why the seizures were happening. After his death, I started writing in my feelings. It became my journal of his death, and how it was affecting me."

Author Frank Fuerst cared for his wife June for seventeen years with Alzheimer's disease. He is the author of ***Alzheimer's Care with Dignity***, and describes daily journaling this way:

"Journalize everything! Date each entry. Writing about your emotions will provide a harmless way of getting rid of negative ones. It will also help to see the positive progression of emotions over time. Putting things in writing clarifies your thoughts. It also makes it easier to set goals, and keep them centermost in one's thoughts. Write about problems that need a solution. As you experiment, write about the solutions and to what degree they might be effective."

Our Daily Connection is a journal to log day-to-day facts and emotions for thirty-one days. Each day has a "Theme of the Day." The theme includes songs, activities, and a food to entice both the caregiver and care receiver to have a good time. There is also a "Tip of the Day" and "Quote of the Day" to guide and inspire you in your daily walk.

Songs:

Music can be soothing and elevate the mood of both the caregiver and care receiver. Many dementia patients who can't take part in a conversation can still sing. Included are several songs for each day's theme. If you don't know any of the songs, then think up one on your own. If you don't know the words to a song, then simply hum—or just make up the lyrics as you go along. It's a guideline, not a rule. Make it a game to remember songs around that theme.

Activities:

"As hypothesized, both depression and decreased cognitive functioning were associated with reduced frequency of enjoyable activity, and the reduction was significantly greater in A.D. [Alzheimer's disease] patients who were depressed than in those who were not depressed, regardless of cognitive level."
~*Rebecca G. Logsdon, PhD, and Linda Teri, PhD*

Neysa Peterson (the co-author of my books on brain illness) opened my mind to the fact that patients with a brain illness experience boredom. Until the later stages, dementia patients are usually able to participate in daily activities. Every care receiver is different, and what they can or will do depends on their mental aptitude, physical ability, and level of interest. Brain illness patients—just like everyone else—need to feel useful and involved. If the need for activity is left unfulfilled, the patient may wander, become fidgety, or act out. Care receivers have different levels of capabilities, so the activity of the day can be modified as needed for your patient. If none of the activities are realistic in your case, then go back to singing and simply leave them out altogether. The best time to start an activity is after breakfast or lunch.

Here are some of the benefits of daily activity for a brain illness patient:
1. They will rest better at night.
2. Activities keep the patient from focusing on what they *can't do*.
3. If you add praise, activities accentuate feelings of self-worth. Keep some gold stars handy.
4. There may be fewer incidents of pacing, restlessness, and wandering.
5. Some activities (like puzzles) can help to stimulate memory.
6. Being active will fuel the patient's appetite.
7. Movement and dancing can strengthen muscles, reduce muscle and joint pain, and increase flexibility.
8. Focusing on and discussing the daily theme may stimulate communication.
9. Some activities have the added benefit of preserving family history and memories.
10. Add helpful chores in with the daily activities.

"Research suggests that creating positive emotional experiences for Alzheimer's patients diminishes distress and behavior problems."

~Pam Belluck

Food:

It can be hard to find something that a patient wants to eat. Adding a food to the theme might help, since it's connected with fun. I'll try to keep it nourishing and not too hard to cook, or you can buy something at the store already prepared.

Author's note:

The "Theme of the Day" is not intended to add work to the caregiver's already crazy day. They are ideas to break up the "same old, same old" routines—for both the caregiver and care receiver. So, whether you simply hum a few bars of the theme songs, or whether you take time to enjoy the songs, activities and food options, it's up to your own discretion. Skip around. Skip a day. It's *your* journal.

If you like the "Theme of the Day", please let me know at joni@jonialdrich.com. Include any ideas you have for other themes. I may use them in the next version!

THIS IS MY COUNTRY

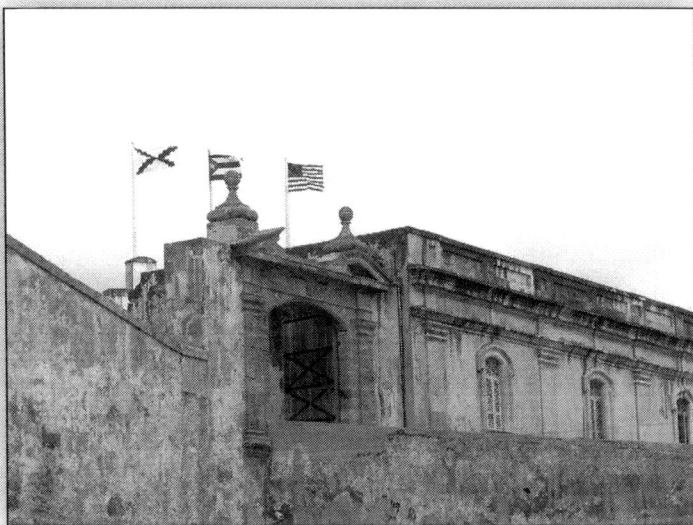

Our flag proudly waves over a fort in Puerto Rico. In 1898, the United States declared war on Spain and, as victor of the war, added Puerto Rico to our country.

~Photo by Joni Aldrich

This is my country! Land of my birth!
This is my country! Grandest on earth!
I pledge thee my allegiance, America, the bold,
For this is my country to have and to hold.

What diff'rence if I hail from North or South,
Or from the East or West?
My heart is filled with love for all of these.
I only know I swell with pride and deep within my breast,
I thrill to see Old Glory paint the breeze.

This is my country! Land of my choice!
This is my country! Hear my proud voice!
I pledge thee my allegiance, America, the bold,
For this is my country to have and to hold.

This is My Country *is an American patriotic folk song composed in 1940. The lyrics are by Don Raye, and the music is by Al Jacobs.*

Date: _____

This is My Country

SONGS:
The National Anthem (lyrics by Francis Scott Key)
America the Beautiful (lyrics by Katharine Lee Bates)
God Bless America (lyrics by Irving Berlin)

ACTIVITIES:
- Have a scavenger hunt in your home to find items with American history.
- Draw and color the American flag.
- Discuss former American presidents and their families.

FOOD:
Apple pie

Tip of the Day:

Caregivers should learn as much as they can about the effects and stages of dementia.

Invest the time necessary to research and understand what is happening with your patient affected by dementia and Alzheimer's disease. There is a lot of information available, and being prepared and proactive is important for the caregiver and care receiver.

Quote of the Day:

"Being willing to change allows you to move from a point of view to a viewing point—a higher, more expansive place, from which you can see both sides."

~ Thomas Crum

Patient notes for today:

Physical or mental changes: _____

_____

_____

_____

Memory changes: _____

_____

_____

_____

Behavioral changes and triggers: _____

_____

_____

_____

Successes: _____

_____

_____

_____

Seizure notes: _____

_____

_____

_____

Medication or doctor notes:_____

_____

_____

_____

Pain level: _____

Energy level: _____

Rest or sleep issues: _____

Speech or word patterns:_____

Overall mood displayed by the patient:

_____

_____

_____

_____

Emotional expressions by the patient:

_____

_____

_____

_____

Caregiver feelings:

Today's feeling is (circle one) a blessing or a released burden:

_____

_____

_____

_____

_____

_____

_____

_____

_____

_____

_____

_____

_____

_____

_____

_____

_____

Other notes:

_____
_____
_____
_____
_____
_____
_____
_____
_____
_____
_____
_____
_____
_____

To do list:

_____
_____
_____
_____
_____
_____
_____
_____
_____
_____
_____
_____
_____
_____
_____
_____

Date: _____

Theme of the Day:
A World of Colors

SONGS:
Blue Bayou (lyrics by Roy Orbison and Joe Melson)
Brown Eyed Girl (lyrics by Van Morrison)
Pink Cadillac (lyrics by Bruce Springsteen)

ACTIVITIES:
- Dance, dance, dance to the music.
- Have an art day. Paint anything you want in many colors.
- Discuss colors and how they affect moods. Red = power and strength; pink = sensitivity and love; yellow/gold = energy; green = harmony in mind, body, and soul; blue = healing and calmness; and violet = spirituality.

FOOD:
A colorful raw vegetable tray.

Tip of the Day:

Document important concerns to discuss with the patient's doctor.

You may have heard that "the devil is in the details." The caregiver plays an important role in the information cycle—especially when the patient has memory issues. Make note of any concerns in this journal, and take it along to the next doctor's visit. Doctors—no matter how good they are—don't read minds.

Quote of the Day:

"It's the little details that are vital.
Little things make big things happen."

~ John Wooden

Patient notes for today:

Physical or mental changes: _____

_____

_____

_____

Memory changes: _____

_____

_____

_____

Behavioral changes and triggers: _____

_____

_____

_____

Successes: _____

_____

_____

Challenges: _____

_____

_____

Seizure notes: _____

_____

_____

Medication or doctor notes:_____

_____

_____

Pain level: _____

Energy level: _____

Rest or sleep issues: _____

Speech or word patterns:_____

Overall mood displayed by the patient:

_____
_____
_____
_____

Emotional expressions by the patient:

_____
_____
_____
_____

Caregiver feelings:

Today's feeling is (circle one) a **blessing** or a released **burden:**

_____
_____
_____
_____
_____
_____
_____
_____
_____
_____
_____
_____
_____
_____
_____
_____

Other notes:

To do list:

ARMED FORCES AND HEROES

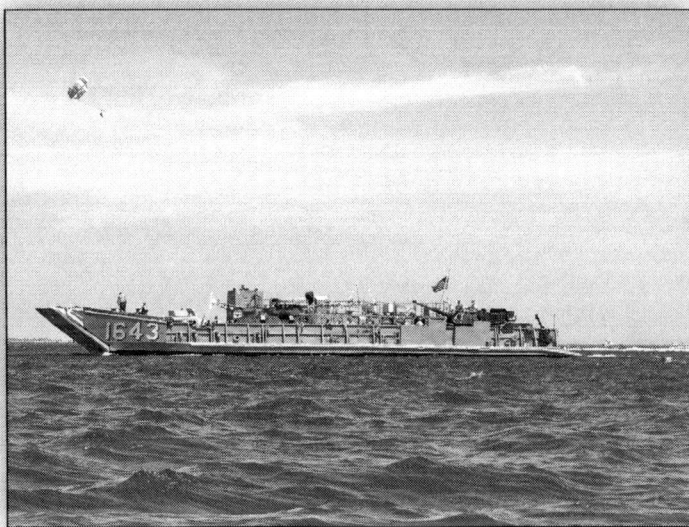

A troop hauler drops off its cargo of soldiers on a beach in North Carolina. The boat was just out for maneuvers, but this looks more like a scene from World War II!

~*Photo by Joni Aldrich*

From the Halls of Montezuma,
To the shores of Tripoli;
We fight our country's battles
In the air, on land, and sea.
First to fight for right and freedom,
And to keep our honor clean.
We are proud to claim the title
Of United States Marine.

The **Marines' Hymn** *is the official hymn of the United States Marine Corps. It is the oldest official song in the United States military.*

Date: _____

Armed Forces and Heroes

SONGS:

Anchor's Away (lyrics by Alfred Hart Miles)

The U. S. Air Force ("Wild Blue Yonder", lyrics by Robert Crawford)

Marine's Hymn (lyrics were popular phrases; actual author unknown)

The Army Goes Rolling Along (lyrics by Edmund L. Gruber)

ACTIVITIES:

- Discuss each branch of our nation's armed services. Don't forget the Coast Guard!
- If either the caregiver or care receiver is a veteran, talk about what you *liked* about being in the service—such as the camaraderie between fellow soldiers.
- Talk about famous generals from George Washington to George S. Patton.

FOOD:

Chicken in water is a healthy canned food. Pretend that it's K-rations.

Tip of the Day:

Caregivers are the un-sung heroes behind every fight for life.

It's rare that anyone takes care of the caregiver. If you get sick, who will take care of the patient? Don't forget to take your medicine, go to doctor's appointments, eat right, and get enough rest.

Quote of the Day:

"A hero is an ordinary individual who finds the strength to persevere and endure in spite of overwhelming obstacles."

~ Christopher Reeve

Patient notes for today:

Physical or mental changes: _____

_____

_____

_____

Memory changes: _____

_____

_____

_____

Behavioral changes and triggers: _____

_____

_____

_____

Successes: _____

_____

_____

Challenges: _____

_____

_____

Seizure notes: _____

_____

_____

Medication or doctor notes:_____

_____

_____

Pain level: _____

Energy level: _____

Rest or sleep issues: _____

Speech or word patterns:_____

Overall mood displayed by the patient:

_____
_____
_____
_____

Emotional expressions by the patient:

_____
_____
_____
_____

Caregiver feelings:

Today's feeling is (circle one) a **blessing** or a released **burden**:

_____
_____
_____
_____
_____
_____
_____
_____
_____
_____
_____
_____
_____
_____
_____
_____

Other notes:

To do list:

Date: _____

Marching to Victory

SONGS:

When the Saints Go Marching In (lyrics by Katharine Purvis)

I Love a Parade (lyrics by Harold Arlen)

Seventy-six Trombones (lyrics by Meredith Willson)

ACTIVITIES:

- Set up your own parade, and march around for great exercise.
- Talk about the different parts of a parade (for example: bands, floats, horses). Which do you like the best?
- Watch a musical, or go to the symphony.

FOOD:

Turkey (in honor of the Macy's Thanksgiving Day parade).

Tip of the Day:

If the patient is physically able, try to schedule daily exercise.

Exercise may help improve both the brain-related symptoms and overall quality of life. Studies have shown that physically active people exhibit higher levels of cognitive functioning than inactive people. The theory is that physically active people have a "cognitive reserve" that is used when other areas of the brain are damaged.

Quote of the Day:

"Physical fitness is not only one of the most important keys to a healthy body, it is the basis of dynamic and creative intellectual activity."

~ John F. Kennedy

Patient notes for today:

Physical or mental changes: _____

_____

_____

_____

Memory changes: _____

_____

_____

_____

Behavioral changes and triggers: _____

_____

_____

_____

Successes: _____

_____

_____

Challenges: _____

_____

_____

Seizure notes: _____

_____

_____

Medication or doctor notes:_____

_____

_____

Pain level: _____

Energy level: _____

Rest or sleep issues: _____

Speech or word patterns:_____

Overall mood displayed by the patient:

_____

_____

_____

_____

Emotional expressions by the patient:

_____

_____

_____

_____

Caregiver feelings:

Today's feeling is (circle one) a blessing or a released burden:

_____

_____

_____

_____

_____

_____

_____

_____

_____

_____

_____

_____

_____

_____

_____

_____

Other notes:

_____
_____
_____
_____
_____
_____
_____
_____
_____
_____
_____
_____
_____
_____

To do list:

_____
_____
_____
_____
_____
_____
_____
_____
_____
_____
_____
_____
_____
_____
_____

CITY OF LIGHTS

This picture of a castle lit up at night was taken in the Caribbean—not in Ireland. It was a beautiful sight—regardless of where it was! A city glowing at night (such as San Francisco) reminds you of a holiday lightshow.

~Photo by Joni Aldrich

Here are some of the most beautiful cities at night in the United States (according to Trip Advisor):

- ✓ Las Vegas
- ✓ Chicago
- ✓ New York City
- ✓ Seattle

Date: _____

City of Lights

SONGS:

Chicago (lyrics by Fred Fisher)

Kansas City (lyrics by Jerry Leiber and Mike Stoller)

New York, New York (lyrics by Fred Ebb)

ACTIVITIES:
- Talk about the big cities you've visited around the world.
- Review a map of different countries, and point out the capital cities.
- Look for photographs of different cities. Make a collage. You get extra points for night photos.

FOOD:
Steak

Tip of the Day:

Each person has his or her own "library" of experiences.

The distant memories of the care receiver may yield some wonderful family history to store for future generations, even if the patient's short-term memory is affected. Once the golden opportunity of experience is lost, it may be lost forever.

Quote of the Day:

**"I embrace emerging experience. I participate in discovery.
I am a butterfly. I am not a butterfly collector.
I want the experience of the butterfly."**

~ William Stafford

Patient notes for today:

Physical or mental changes: _____

_____

_____

_____

Memory changes: _____

_____

_____

_____

Behavioral changes and triggers: _____

_____

_____

_____

Successes: _____

_____

_____

Challenges: _____

_____

_____

Seizure notes: _____

_____

_____

Medication or doctor notes: _____

_____

_____

Pain level: _____

Energy level: _____

Rest or sleep issues: _____

Speech or word patterns: _____

Overall mood displayed by the patient:

_____
_____
_____
_____

Emotional expressions by the patient:

_____
_____
_____
_____

Caregiver feelings:

Today's feeling is (circle one) a **blessing** or a released **burden**:

_____
_____
_____
_____
_____
_____
_____
_____
_____
_____
_____
_____
_____
_____
_____
_____
_____
_____

Other notes:

To do list:

Date: _____

The States of Our Union

SONGS:

Georgia on My Mind (lyrics by Stuart Gorrell)

The Yellow Rose of Texas (author unknown)

Blue Hawaii (written by Leo Robin and Ralph Rainger)

ACTIVITIES:
- See how many of the states you can name.
- Talk about state capitals, state flowers and state birds.
- Look at a map of your state. Which places have you visited?

FOOD:
Peaches

Tip of the Day:

**Reasoning and logic usually doesn't work
with a brain illness patient.**

Your first instinct is to reason. This may lead to frustration, because the patient may be unable to follow lengthy explanations. Trial and error will require all of your patience and people skills. If you want to try reasoning first, use simple, straightforward language.

Quote of the Day:

**"Reasoning draws a conclusion, but does not make the conclusion
certain, unless the mind discovers it by the path of experience."**

~ Roger Bacon

Patient notes for today:

Physical or mental changes: _____

_____

_____

_____

Memory changes: _____

_____

_____

_____

Behavioral changes and triggers: _____

_____

_____

_____

Successes: _____

_____

_____

Challenges: _____

_____

_____

Seizure notes: _____

_____

_____

Medication or doctor notes:_____

_____

_____

Pain level: _____

Energy level: _____

Rest or sleep issues: _____

Speech or word patterns:_____

Overall mood displayed by the patient:

_____
_____
_____
_____

Emotional expressions by the patient:

_____
_____
_____
_____

Caregiver feelings:

Today's feeling is (circle one) a blessing or a released burden:

_____
_____
_____
_____
_____
_____
_____
_____
_____
_____
_____
_____
_____
_____
_____

Other notes:

To do list:

MAMMA MIA: THAT'S ITALIAN

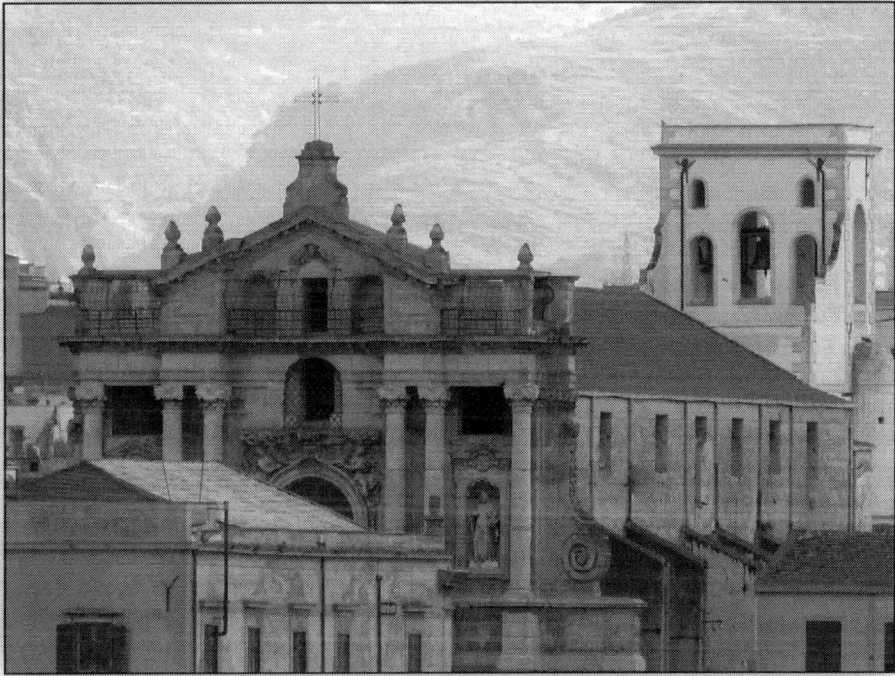

These buildings are classically Italian, and illustrate the beauty found throughout the Italian island of Sicily.

~*Photo by Joni Aldrich*

Listed below are the top ten countries to visit (according to Lonely Planet):

1. Albania
2. Brazil
3. Cape Verde (an island off the coast of Africa)
4. Panama
5. Bulgaria
6. Vanuatu

7. Italy
8. Tanzania
9. Syria
10. Japan

Date: _____

Mamma Mia: That's Italian

SONGS:

That's Amore (lyrics by Jack Brooks; wait—that name isn't Italian)

Mamma Mia (lyrics by Benny Andersson and Björn Ulvaeus)

O Sole Mio (lyrics by Giovanni Capurro—now that's Italian)

ACTIVITIES:

- Watch (what else?) the movie *Mamma Mia*.
- Make your favorite Italian food. Pizza is fun and easy!
- What Italian words do you know? Here are some examples:

    Ciao (Hi)   Arrivederci (Goodbye)

    Si (Yes)   Bello (Beautiful)   Grazie (Thank You)

FOOD:

Italian (choose your favorites)

Tip of the Day:

**Adjust your communication style to the
patient's changing comprehension.**

If you're having difficulty communicating with the patient, try to develop signals related to their basic needs, such as hunger, thirst, and boredom. Document successful patterns in this journal.

Quote of the Day:

**"The more elaborate our means of communication,
the less we communicate."**

~Joseph Priestley

Patient notes for today:

Physical or mental changes: _____

_____

_____

_____

Memory changes: _____

_____

_____

_____

Behavioral changes and triggers: _____

_____

_____

_____

Successes: _____

_____

_____

Challenges: _____

_____

_____

Seizure notes: _____

_____

_____

Medication or doctor notes: _____

_____

_____

_____

Pain level: _____

Energy level: _____

Rest or sleep issues: _____

Speech or word patterns: _____

Overall mood displayed by the patient:

_____

_____

_____

_____

Emotional expressions by the patient:

_____

_____

_____

_____

Caregiver feelings:

Today's feeling is (circle one) a blessing or a released burden:

_____

_____

_____

_____

_____

_____

_____

_____

_____

_____

_____

_____

_____

_____

_____

_____

Other notes:

_____
_____
_____
_____
_____
_____
_____
_____
_____
_____
_____
_____
_____

To do list:

_____
_____
_____
_____
_____
_____
_____
_____
_____
_____
_____
_____
_____

Date: _____

Parlez-vous Français: International

SONGS:

I Love Paris (lyrics by Nat King Cole)

London Bridge (Unknown)

My Wild Irish Rose (lyrics by Chauncey Olcott)

ACTIVITIES:

- Identify countries on a globe or map, and discuss a little about each one.
- Create a collage of pictures that you've taken (or found) of other countries.
- Discuss the countries that border the United States.

FOOD:

Croissants

Tip of the Day:

Be an advocate for comfort and safety in the home.

Continually adapting to the patient's current status is necessary, but may be challenging. If the patient is showing signs of instability while standing or walking, they may need constant supervision. In some ways, it may seem that you're childproofing the house—only the patient is much taller!

Quote of the Day:

"Prepare and prevent, don't repair and repent."

~ Author Unknown

Patient notes for today:

Physical or mental changes: _____

_____

_____

_____

Memory changes: _____

_____

_____

_____

Behavioral changes and triggers: _____

_____

_____

_____

Successes: _____

_____

_____

Challenges: _____

_____

_____

Seizure notes: _____

_____

_____

Medication or doctor notes: _____

_____

_____

_____

Pain level: _____

Energy level: _____

Rest or sleep issues: _____

Speech or word patterns: _____

Overall mood displayed by the patient:

_____

_____

_____

_____

Emotional expressions by the patient:

_____

_____

_____

_____

Caregiver feelings:

Today's feeling is (circle one) a **blessing** or a released **burden**:

_____

_____

_____

_____

_____

_____

_____

_____

_____

_____

_____

_____

_____

_____

_____

Other notes:

_____
_____
_____
_____
_____
_____
_____
_____
_____
_____
_____
_____

To do list:

_____
_____
_____
_____
_____
_____
_____
_____
_____
_____
_____
_____
_____
_____

Date: _____

SONGS:

It's Been a Hard Days Night (lyrics by John Lennon)

Yellow Submarine (lyrics by Paul McCartney)

I Want to Hold Your Hand (lyrics by John Lennon and Paul McCartney)

ACTIVITIES:
- Name the four members of The Beatles. Who was your favorite?
- Discuss the history of the band, and how they became famous. (Hint: The Ed Sullivan Show)
- Dance to the original rock and roll band.

FOOD:
Submarine sandwiches

Tip of the Day:

**Even if the care receiver seems unresponsive,
continue to offer soothing words and comfort.**

A dementia patient still thrives on human interaction. If treated unfairly or ignored, the care receiver may feel rejected and lonely. Treat the patient the way that you would want to be treated.

Quote of the Day:

**"Respect for ourselves guides our morals;
respect for others guides our manners."**

~ Laurence Sterne

Patient notes for today:

Physical or mental changes: _____

_____

_____

_____

Memory changes: _____

_____

_____

_____

Behavioral changes and triggers: _____

_____

_____

_____

Successes: _____

_____

_____

Challenges: _____

_____

_____

Seizure notes: _____

_____

_____

Medication or doctor notes:_____

_____

_____

_____

Pain level: _____

Energy level: _____

Rest or sleep issues: _____

Speech or word patterns:_____

Overall mood displayed by the patient:

_____

_____

_____

_____

Emotional expressions by the patient:

_____

_____

_____

_____

Caregiver feelings:

Today's feeling is (circle one) a blessing or a released burden:

_____

_____

_____

_____

_____

_____

_____

_____

_____

_____

_____

_____

_____

_____

_____

_____

Other notes:

To do list:

BOATS

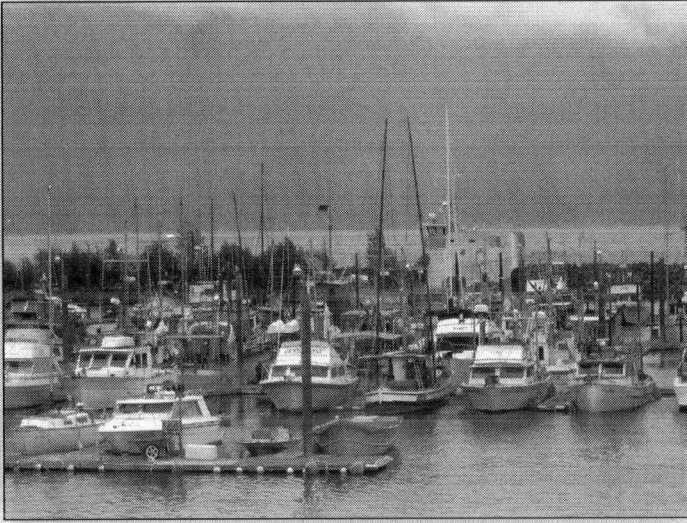

This view of fishing boats at rest was taken in Ketchikan, Alaska. There's just nothing as peaceful as a safe harbor.

~Photo by Joni Aldrich

Michael Row the Boat Ashore is a spiritual that combines religious expression with daily labor. The more popular theory is that Michael is the archangel Michael, who is being called on to help when the rowing gets tough. The song's popularity soared after Harry Belafonte recorded it. Although there are many different versions, the more familiar modern-era lines are from Pete Seeger's version:

> "Jordan's river is deep and wide, hallelujah.
> Meet my mother on the other side, hallelujah.
> Jordan's river is chilly and cold, hallelujah.
> Chills the body, but not the soul, hallelujah."

Date: _____

Theme of the Day:
Boats

SONGS:

Michael Row the Boat Ashore (traditional spiritual)

Row, Row, Row Your Boat (from a nursery rhyme)

Boat Drinks (lyrics by Jimmy Buffet)

ACTIVITIES:

- Discuss the different types of boats (for example: tug, sailboat, freighter, yacht, houseboat).
- Make fruity, refreshing boat drinks (minus the alcohol).
- Float a boat (plastic or remote control) in a bathtub, lake or pond.

FOOD:
Shrimp

Tip of the Day:

**No matter how hard you try, mistakes
(hopefully minor ones) will happen.**

Just as the care receiver is human, the caregiver is human, too. Each in turn must learn the value of forgiveness. Accept that a mistake was made, and move on. Apologies are always good medicine.

Quote of the Day:

**"A man should never be ashamed to own that he
is wrong, which is but saying in other words that
he is wiser today than he was yesterday."**

~ Alexander Pope

Patient notes for today:

Physical or mental changes: _____

_____

_____

_____

Memory changes: _____

_____

_____

_____

Behavioral changes and triggers: _____

_____

_____

_____

Successes: _____

_____

_____

Challenges: _____

_____

_____

Seizure notes: _____

_____

_____

Medication or doctor notes: _____

_____

_____

_____

Pain level: _____

Energy level: _____

Rest or sleep issues: _____

Speech or word patterns: _____

Overall mood displayed by the patient:

_____

_____

_____

_____

Emotional expressions by the patient:

_____

_____

_____

_____

Caregiver feelings:

Today's feeling is (circle one) a blessing or a released burden:

_____

_____

_____

_____

_____

_____

_____

_____

_____

_____

_____

_____

_____

_____

_____

_____

_____

Other notes:

_____
_____
_____
_____
_____
_____
_____
_____
_____
_____
_____
_____
_____

To do list:

_____
_____
_____
_____
_____
_____
_____
_____
_____
_____
_____
_____
_____
_____
_____

Date: _____

Trains

SONGS:

I've Been Working on the Railroad (American folk song)

Chattanooga Choo Choo (lyrics by Mack Gordon)

Night Train to Memphis (written by Bradley, Hughes and Smith)

ACTIVITIES:
- Plan your own train route around the places that you'd like to visit.
- Discuss the different sections of a train (for example: engine, caboose, dining car).
- Put up a train set. If you don't have a real one, make one out of cardboard shoeboxes.

FOOD:

Johnny Cash chicken casserole (make your personal favorite and rename it)

Tip of the Day:

As you listen and respond to your care receiver,
always remain flexible, patient, and calm.

Don't argue, or try to emphatically convince the patient. Acknowledge requests, and respond to them. Look for the need behind each statement and behavior.

Quote of the Day:

"Adopt the pace of nature; her secret is patience."

~ Ralph Waldo Emerson

Patient notes for today:

Physical or mental changes: _____

_____

_____

_____

Memory changes: _____

_____

_____

_____

Behavioral changes and triggers: _____

_____

_____

_____

Successes: _____

_____

_____

Challenges: _____

_____

_____

Seizure notes: _____

_____

_____

Medication or doctor notes: _____

_____

_____

_____

Pain level: _____

Energy level: _____

Rest or sleep issues: _____

Speech or word patterns: _____

Overall mood displayed by the patient:

_____

_____

_____

_____

Emotional expressions by the patient:

_____

_____

_____

_____

Caregiver feelings:

Today's feeling is (circle one) a blessing or a released burden:

_____

_____

_____

_____

_____

_____

_____

_____

_____

_____

_____

_____

_____

_____

_____

_____

_____

Other notes:

To do list:

IT'S A PIRATE'S LIFE FOR ME

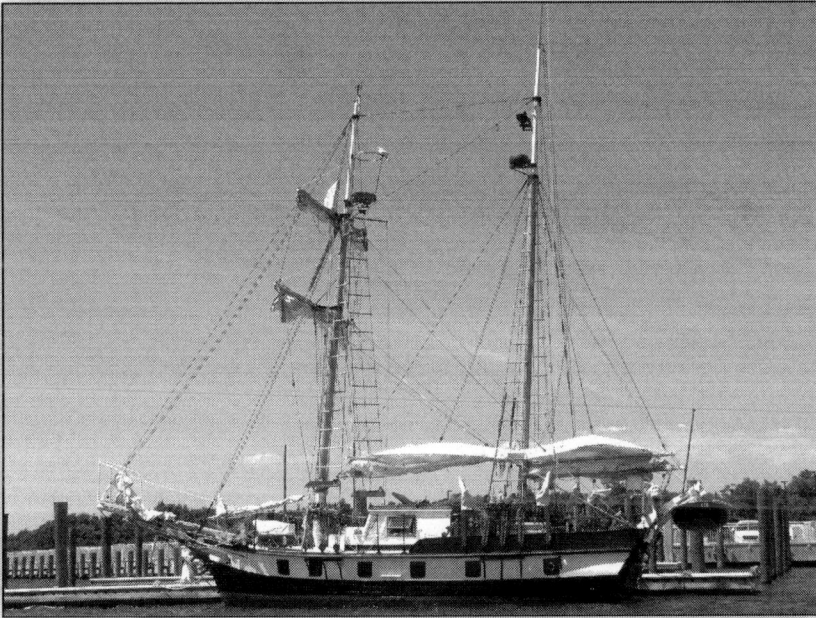

In my hometown of Beaufort, North Carolina, this is Sinbad the Pirate's ship. It was moored at dock on this sunny day. I guess the pirates were resting. Aaaarrrrgggghhhh!

~Photo by Joni Aldrich

A pirate's story from the North Carolina coast:
One of the most beautiful coastal areas in the United States stretches from Cape Hatteras to Wilmington, North Carolina. Blackbeard lived, pillaged, and died in these parts. In 1996, an ancient shipwreck found in Beaufort Inlet was identified as the Queen Anne's Revenge—Blackbeard's flagship.

"Arrr, he's like a duck without wings! We'll close for the kill, and then board her. And I'll dangle Uncle Harry from the foreyard!"

~Blackbeard, the Pirate (source unknown)

Date: _____

Theme of the Day:

It's a Pirate's Life for Me

SONGS:

Yo Ho—A Pirate's Life for Me (lyrics by Xavier Atencio)

Blow the Man Down (old sea shanty)

Yo Ho Ho and a Bottle of Rum (lyrics by Young Ewing Allison)

ACTIVITIES:

- Have fun practicing your pirate language, including:

  Aye! (Yes)

  Aaaarrrrgggghhhh! (Expression of discontent or disgust.)

  Ahoy! (Hello)

  Ahoy, Matey (Hello, my friend!)

  Ahoy, me hearties! (Hello, my friends!)

  All hand hoay! (All hands on deck.)

- Talk about interesting pirates, such as Blackbeard, Anne Bonney, and even Jack Sparrow!

- Draw a treasure map. Hide and seek a treasure chest!

FOOD:

Dried beans (pirate ship rations—cooked, of course)

Tip of the Day:

Don't lie to the patient—not even little white lies.

Lying could lead to mistrust and paranoia from your care receiver. These are not problems that you want to have to overcome.

Quote of the Day:

"Lying is done with words and also with silence."

~Adrienne Rich

Patient notes for today:

Physical or mental changes: _____

_____

_____

_____

Memory changes: _____

_____

_____

_____

Behavioral changes and triggers: _____

_____

_____

_____

Successes: _____

_____

_____

Challenges: _____

_____

_____

Seizure notes: _____

_____

_____

Medication or doctor notes: _____

_____

_____

_____

Pain level: _____

Energy level: _____

Rest or sleep issues: _____

Speech or word patterns: _____

Overall mood displayed by the patient:

_____

_____

_____

_____

Emotional expressions by the patient:

_____

_____

_____

_____

Caregiver feelings:

Today's feeling is (circle one) a **blessing** or a released **burden:**

_____

_____

_____

_____

_____

_____

_____

_____

_____

_____

_____

_____

_____

_____

_____

_____

Other notes:

To do list:

Date: _____

SONGS:

Don't Worry, Be Happy (lyrics by Bobby McFerrin)

Tiptoe Through the Tulips (Tiny Tim style; lyrics by Al Dubin)

Ahab the Arab (written and recorded by Ray Stevens)

ACTIVITIES:
- Listen to "clean" comics.
- Watch some classic comedy movies or cartoons.
- Discuss different comedians, and why you like them. Start with the old classics, such as Lucille Ball.

FOOD:
Ham

Tip of the Day:

Effective communication is composed of many different attributes.

Communication includes listening, interpreting, understanding the underlying emotions, identifying the need, and reassuring the patient through validation of their feelings.

Quote of the Day:

"Everything becomes a little different as soon as it is spoken out loud."

~ Hermann Hesse

Patient notes for today:

Physical or mental changes: _____

_____

_____

_____

Memory changes: _____

_____

_____

_____

Behavioral changes and triggers: _____

_____

_____

_____

Successes: _____

_____

_____

Challenges: _____

_____

_____

Seizure notes: _____

_____

_____

Medication or doctor notes: _____

_____

_____

_____

Pain level: _____

Energy level: _____

Rest or sleep issues: _____

Speech or word patterns: _____

Overall mood displayed by the patient:

_____
_____
_____
_____

Emotional expressions by the patient:

_____
_____
_____
_____

Caregiver feelings:

Today's feeling is (circle one) a **blessing** or a released **burden:**

_____
_____
_____
_____
_____
_____
_____
_____
_____
_____
_____
_____
_____
_____
_____
_____

Other notes:

To do list:

CALYPSO

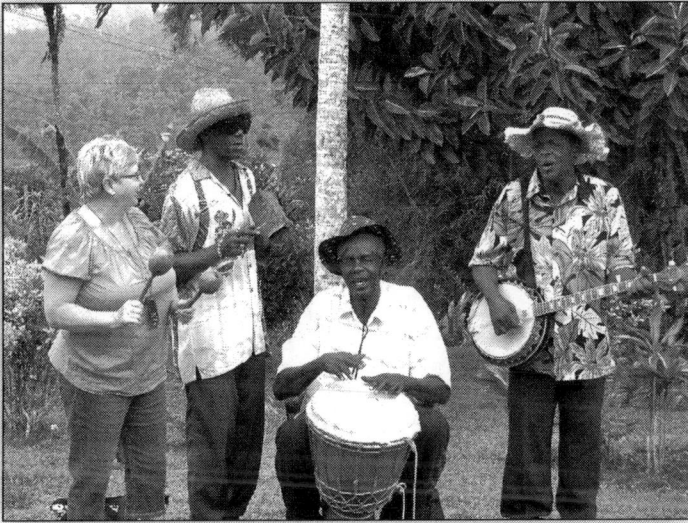

A calypso band in Grenada gets a little help from a friendly tourist. It was fun for everyone.

~Photo by Joni Aldrich

The history of calypso music is fascinating. At first, the musicians made their own instruments, often out of the bottoms (the pans) of metal shipping containers, paint cans, and garbage cans. During World War II, empty 55-gallon oil drums became widely used. The more recent instrument makers perfected their technique, making and selling pan drums that could play an entire scale. The steel drum is the only acoustic (non-electric) instrument invented in the twentieth century.

"Aruba, Jamaica ooo I wanna take you
Bermuda, Bahama come on pretty mama..."

Date: _____

Calypso

SONGS:

Day-O, The Banana Boat Song (Jamaican folk song)

Kokomo (written by The Beach Boys, but Mike Love added: "Aruba, Jamaica")

One World, One Love (written and recorded by Bob Marley)

ACTIVITIES:

- Reggae dance around the house.
- Discuss the different Caribbean islands, and what makes them so beautiful.
- Practice a laid-back lifestyle!

FOOD:

Johnnycake (cornmeal flatbread)

Mix together one-half cup of flour, one cup of cornmeal, one tsp. sugar, one tsp. salt, one lightly beaten egg, one cup of hot milk, and one tbsp. shortening. Fry the "cakes" on a hot, greased griddle or iron skillet.

Tip of the Day:

Add a little fun to every day with your care receiver.

Prevent the doldrums by planning a weekly activity sheet and simple lesson plans. Your daily plan should include the title, objective, materials needed, and feedback on how the activity was accepted by the patient. Happiness is something that should happen every day.

Quote of the Day:

"People rarely succeed unless they have fun in what they are doing."

~Dale Carnegie

Patient notes for today:

Physical or mental changes: _____

_____

_____

_____

Memory changes: _____

_____

_____

_____

Behavioral changes and triggers: _____

_____

_____

_____

Successes: _____

_____

_____

Challenges: _____

_____

_____

Seizure notes: _____

_____

_____

Medication or doctor notes:_____

_____

_____

_____

Pain level: _____

Energy level: _____

Rest or sleep issues: _____

Speech or word patterns:_____

Overall mood displayed by the patient:

_____

_____

_____

_____

Emotional expressions by the patient:

_____

_____

_____

_____

Caregiver feelings:

Today's feeling is (circle one) a blessing or a released burden:

_____

_____

_____

_____

_____

_____

_____

_____

_____

_____

_____

_____

_____

_____

_____

Other notes:

To do list:

Date: _____

Fruits of Life

SONGS:

Blueberry Hill (lyrics by Larry Stock)

Don't Sit Under the Apple Tree (by Stept, Brown and Tobias)

Lemon Tree (lyrics by Will Holt)

ACTIVITIES:

- Make a list of your favorite fruits, and discuss how they grow (on a bush, plant or tree). Hint: "Lemon tree very pretty..."
- Draw and paint the fruits on your list. Make it a "still life" work of free-style art.
- Get some fresh exotic fruits, and have a taste test (for example, passion fruit, star fruit, kumquat, dragon fruit).

FOOD:

Fruit salad

Tip of the Day:

The patient may have forgotten your name, but he or she might still recall the essence of who you are.

You are familiar, and have a close history with the patient. In some cases, they may remember the names of those closest to them, but not the less frequent visitors. What's in a name? Try to remember that your name isn't truly who you are.

Quote of the Day:

"It is surprising how much of memory is built around things unnoticed at the time."

~ Barbara Kingsolver

Patient notes for today:

Physical or mental changes: _____

_____

_____

_____

Memory changes: _____

_____

_____

_____

Behavioral changes and triggers: _____

_____

_____

_____

Successes: _____

_____

_____

Challenges: _____

_____

_____

Seizure notes: _____

_____

_____

Medication or doctor notes: _____

_____

_____

_____

Pain level: _____

Energy level: _____

Rest or sleep issues: _____

Speech or word patterns: _____

Overall mood displayed by the patient:

_____

_____

_____

_____

Emotional expressions by the patient:

_____

_____

_____

_____

Caregiver feelings:

Today's feeling is (circle one) a **blessing** or a released **burden**:

_____

_____

_____

_____

_____

_____

_____

_____

_____

_____

_____

_____

_____

_____

_____

Other notes:

To do list:

GONE FISHING

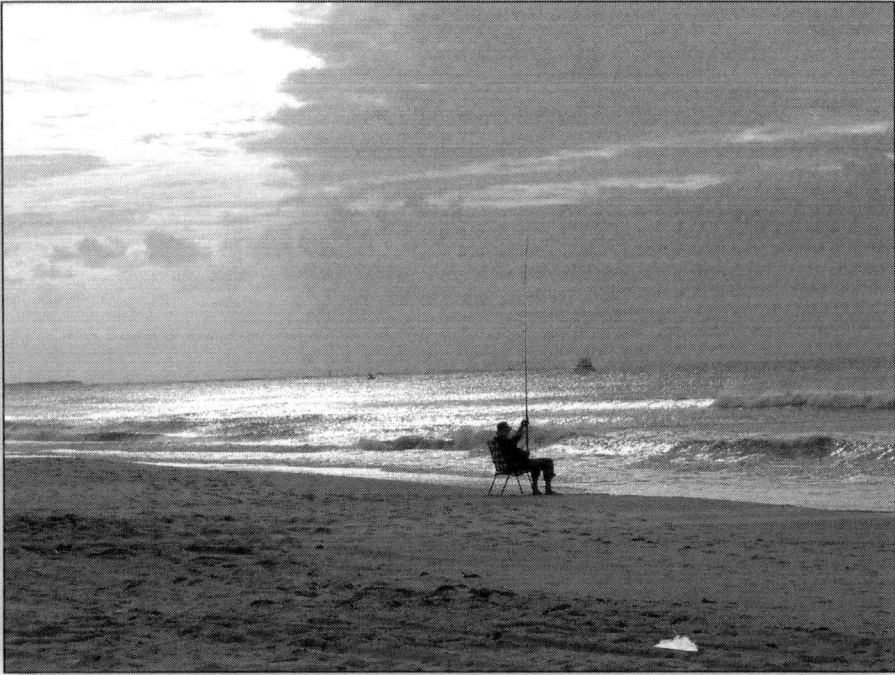

As the sun begins to set, this surf fisherman has a great seat for a sunset show. He seems quite relaxed as he casts his line into the ocean waves off of Atlantic Beach, North Carolina.

~Photo by Joni Aldrich

Gone Fishing (lyrics by Chris Rea)

> I'm gone fishing,
> Sounds crazy I know.
> I know nothing about fishing,
> But just watch me go.

And when my time has come,
I will look back and see,
Peace on the shoreline
That could have been me.

Date: _____

SONGS:

Gone Fishing (there are several versions, but my favorite is by Chris Rea)

Under the Sea (lyrics by Howard Ashman for *The Little Mermaid*)

Flipper (lyrics by William D. "By" Dunham)

ACTIVITIES:
- Watch *Finding Nemo* or *The Little Mermaid*.
- Play the card game: "Go Fish."
- Visit an ocean aquarium, or go to see aquariums at a pet store.

FOOD:
Tuna salad

Tip of the Day:

Use creative diversion techniques to prevent negative activities.

An effective caregiver knows what is best for the patient. If the patient is allergic to peanuts—you have to say "no" to peanuts. Offer an alternative, or use the art of distraction to divert the need. Diversion is one of your most effective tools with a brain illness patient.

Quote of the Day:

"Everything that lives, lives not alone, nor for itself."

~ William Blake

Patient notes for today:

Physical or mental changes: _____

_____

_____

_____

Memory changes: _____

_____

_____

_____

Behavioral changes and triggers: _____

_____

_____

_____

Successes: _____

_____

_____

Challenges: _____

_____

_____

Seizure notes: _____

_____

_____

Medication or doctor notes:_____

_____

_____

_____

Pain level: _____

Energy level: _____

Rest or sleep issues: _____

Speech or word patterns:_____

Overall mood displayed by the patient:

_____
_____
_____
_____

Emotional expressions by the patient:

_____
_____
_____
_____

Caregiver feelings:

Today's feeling is (circle one) a **blessing** or a released **burden**:

_____
_____
_____
_____
_____
_____
_____
_____
_____
_____
_____
_____
_____
_____
_____
_____

Other notes:

To do list:

Date: _____

A Picture's Worth a Thousand Words

SONGS:

Memories (words and music by Bill Strange and Scott Davis)

Time in a Bottle (written and recorded by Jim Croce)

Mona Lisa (written by Ray Evans and Jay Livingston)

ACTIVITIES:
- Make a photo album.
- Get a disposable camera, and let the care receiver take all of the pictures.
- Look at photographs of family members and personal trips, and talk about the happy memories.

FOOD:
Mushrooms

Tip of the Day:

Expect the patient to change—possibly on a daily basis. Learn to change with the change.

There will be days of clarity, and days of not so much clarity. Expect the unexpected; appreciate the good days, and patiently work through the bad days.

Quote of the Day:

"Happy memories become treasures in the heart to pull out on the tough days of adulthood."

~ Charlotte Davis Kasl

Patient notes for today:

Physical or mental changes: _____

_____

_____

_____

Memory changes: _____

_____

_____

_____

Behavioral changes and triggers: _____

_____

_____

_____

Successes: _____

_____

_____

Challenges: _____

_____

_____

Seizure notes: _____

_____

_____

Medication or doctor notes: _____

_____

_____

_____

Pain level: _____

Energy level: _____

Rest or sleep issues: _____

Speech or word patterns: _____

Overall mood displayed by the patient:

_____

_____

_____

_____

Emotional expressions by the patient:

_____

_____

_____

_____

Caregiver feelings:

Today's feeling is (circle one) a **blessing** or a released **burden**:

_____

_____

_____

_____

_____

_____

_____

_____

_____

_____

_____

_____

_____

_____

_____

Other notes:

To do list:

DOWN ON THE FARM

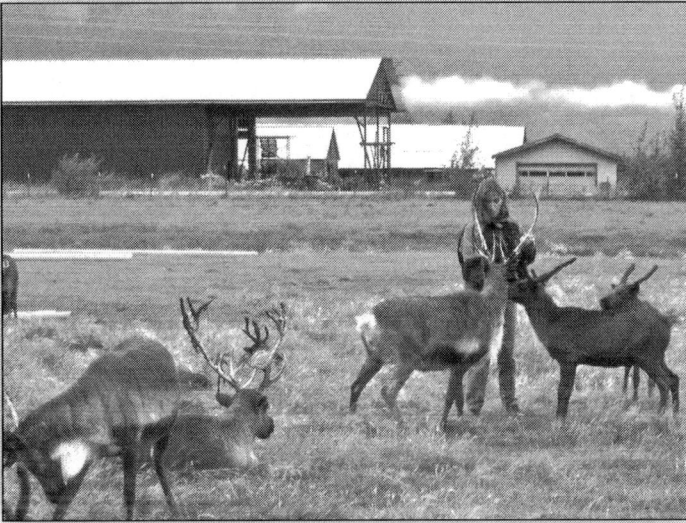

In 2003, the author visited this reindeer farm in Alaska. The reindeers tended to mob any person with a free snack.

~Photo by Gordon Aldrich

Agriculture is a major industry in the United States. As of the last census of agriculture in 2007, there were 2.1 million farms covering an area of 922 million acres (an amazing average of 418 acres per farm). Major crops include: corn, soybeans, wheat, alfalfa, cotton, hay, tobacco, rice, sorghum, and barley. Livestock farmers raise the following: dairy cattle, beef cattle, swine, poultry, and sheep.

Date: _____

Theme of the Day:
Down on the Farm

SONGS:

The Farmer in the Dell (a singing game based on a nursery rhyme)

Old McDonald Had a Farm (an old folk song full of animal sounds)

Green Acres (for the TV show; lyrics by Vic Mizzy)

ACTIVITIES:
- Visit a petting zoo, pet store or farm.
- Put together a puzzle of a farm scene or animals.
- Cut out and sort recipes, then try some of your favorites.

FOOD:
Vegetable soup (use fresh vegetables, if you can)

Tip of the Day:
**Dementia patients need a diet rich in
vitamins, minerals and nutrients.**

Consult with the patient's doctor regarding proper nutrition and supplements. Vitamin E is important, but the correct dosage for each care receiver may be different. Thiamin is beneficial and may help with memory improvement, but should also be given in the correct dosage.

Quote of the Day:
**"Ninety percent of the diseases known to man are
caused by cheap foodstuffs. You are what you eat."**

~ Dr. Victor Lindlahr

Patient notes for today:

Physical or mental changes: _____

_____

_____

_____

Memory changes: _____

_____

_____

_____

Behavioral changes and triggers: _____

_____

_____

_____

Successes: _____

_____

_____

Challenges: _____

_____

_____

Seizure notes: _____

_____

_____

Medication or doctor notes: _____

_____

_____

_____

Pain level: _____

Energy level: _____

Rest or sleep issues: _____

Speech or word patterns: _____

Overall mood displayed by the patient:

_____

_____

_____

_____

Emotional expressions by the patient:

_____

_____

_____

_____

Caregiver feelings:

Today's feeling is (circle one) a **blessing** or a released **burden**:

_____

_____

_____

_____

_____

_____

_____

_____

_____

_____

_____

_____

_____

_____

_____

_____

_____

Other notes:

To do list:

Date: _____

Theme of the Day:

Commercials to Remember

SONGS:

Plop! Plop! Fizz! Fizz! (commercial for Alka-Seltzer)

I'd Like to Buy the World a Coke (commercial for The Coca-Cola Company)

You Deserve a Break Today (commercial for McDonalds)

ACTIVITIES:

- Sing your favorite commercial jingles.
- While you're watching TV, talk about the commercials.
- Clip, sort and store coupons for the grocery store.

FOOD:

Take a field trip to McDonalds.

Tip of the Day:

Repetitively affirm good, healthful behavior.

It's important to say "thank you" for activity that you once took for granted. If the patient helps to put away the clothes—even if they're in the wrong place—offer a word of thanks for the help. This may seem small to you, but it's huge to the patient.

Quote of the Day:

"Silent gratitude isn't much use to anyone."

~Gladys Browyn Stern

Patient notes for today:

Physical or mental changes: _____

_____

_____

_____

Memory changes: _____

_____

_____

_____

Behavioral changes and triggers: _____

_____

_____

_____

Successes: _____

_____

_____

Challenges: _____

_____

_____

Seizure notes: _____

_____

_____

Medication or doctor notes: _____

_____

_____

_____

Pain level: _____

Energy level: _____

Rest or sleep issues: _____

Speech or word patterns: _____

Overall mood displayed by the patient:

_____

_____

_____

_____

Emotional expressions by the patient:

_____

_____

_____

_____

Caregiver feelings:

Today's feeling is (circle one) a **blessing** or a released **burden**:

_____

_____

_____

_____

_____

_____

_____

_____

_____

_____

_____

_____

_____

_____

_____

_____

Other notes:

To do list:

MOTHER NATURE

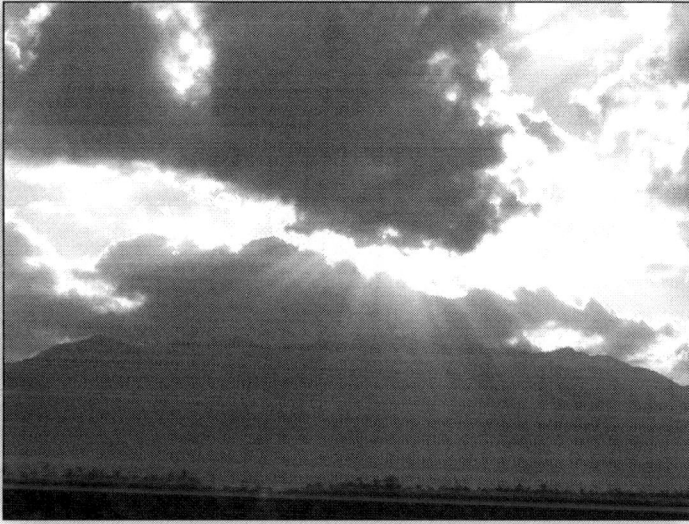

Mother Nature shines brightly through the cloudy sky, and illuminates this stately mountain range.

~*Photo by Joni Aldrich*

Nature – the Gentlest Mother is, poem by Emily Dickinson

> Nature the gentlest mother is,
> Impatient of no child.
> The feeblest or the waywardest,
> Her admonition mild.
>
> How fair her conversation;
> A summer afternoon.
> Her household, her assembly,
> And when the sun go down.

With infinite affection,
And infiniter care.
Her golden finger on her lip,
Wills silence everywhere.

Date: _____

Theme of the Day:

Mother Nature

SONGS:

Over the Rainbow (lyrics by E.Y. Harburg)

You Are My Sunshine (by Jimmie Davis and Charles Mitchell)

Twinkle, Twinkle, Little Star (based on "The Star" by Jane Taylor)

ACTIVITIES:
- Draw a colorful rainbow.
- Watch The Wizard of Oz.
- Discuss star formations like The Little Dipper.

FOOD:
Rainbow pancakes (pancake mix with food coloring).

Tip of the Day:

Choose comforting topics to discuss.

Talk about the patient's childhood, family, and work career. My mother recently offered some wonderful memories about her family that I didn't know. These are gifts to be treasured.

Quote of the Day:

**"Oh the comfort, the inexpressible comfort of feeling
safe with a person, having neither to weigh thoughts nor
measure words, but pouring them all right out, just as
they are – chaff and grain together – certain that a faithful
hand will take and sift them, keep what is worth keeping,
and with the breath of kindness blow the rest away."**

~Dinah Mulock

Patient notes for today:

Physical or mental changes: _____

_____

_____

_____

Memory changes: _____

_____

_____

_____

Behavioral changes and triggers: _____

_____

_____

_____

Successes: _____

_____

_____

Challenges: _____

_____

_____

Seizure notes: _____

_____

_____

Medication or doctor notes:_____

_____

_____

_____

Pain level: _____

Energy level: _____

Rest or sleep issues: _____

Speech or word patterns:_____

Overall mood displayed by the patient:

_____
_____
_____
_____

Emotional expressions by the patient:

_____
_____
_____
_____

Caregiver feelings:

Today's feeling is (circle one) a blessing or a released burden:

_____
_____
_____
_____
_____
_____
_____
_____
_____
_____
_____
_____
_____
_____
_____

Other notes:

_____
_____
_____
_____
_____
_____
_____
_____
_____
_____
_____
_____
_____

To do list:

_____
_____
_____
_____
_____
_____
_____
_____
_____
_____
_____
_____
_____
_____

Date: _____

Theme of the Day:

A Little Rain Must Fall

SONGS:

Singin' in the Rain (lyrics by Arthur Freed)

My Favorite Things (lyrics by Oscar Hammerstein II)

It's Raining, It's Pouring (nursery rhyme)

ACTIVITIES:
- Go swimming.
- Draw and color a tree on construction paper. Add a leaf for each of your favorite things. Glue them to the tree.
- Do some things that you usually only do on rainy days. Cocoa anyone?

FOOD:
Oatmeal (warmth for a rainy day)

Tip of the Day:

Bathing may become a battle. Try to establish a routine.

Don't interrupt the routine unless absolutely necessary—not even for visitors. Lay out everything that you'll need in advance. Transform the bathing area into a "day at the spa" atmosphere (minus the candles).

Quote of the Day:

"Rain is grace; rain is the sky condescending to the earth. Without rain, there would be no life."

~John Updike

Patient notes for today:

Physical or mental changes: _____

_____

_____

_____

Memory changes: _____

_____

_____

_____

Behavioral changes and triggers: _____

_____

_____

_____

Successes: _____

_____

_____

Challenges: _____

_____

_____

Seizure notes: _____

_____

_____

Medication or doctor notes: _____

_____

_____

_____

Pain level: _____

Energy level: _____

Rest or sleep issues: _____

Speech or word patterns: _____

Overall mood displayed by the patient:

_____
_____
_____
_____

Emotional expressions by the patient:

_____
_____
_____
_____

Caregiver feelings:

Today's feeling is (circle one) a **blessing** or a released **burden**:

_____
_____
_____
_____
_____
_____
_____
_____
_____
_____
_____
_____
_____
_____
_____

Other notes:

To do list:

Date: _____

SONGS:

Mister Sandman (written by Pat Ballard)

Dream Lover (written and recorded by Bobby Darin)

Beautiful Dreamer (written by Stephen Foster)

ACTIVITIES:

- Play "blindfold" (as long as it doesn't bother the patient); try to identify objects by touch or feel.
- Set up a tent with a bed sheet, and camp in.
- Chore day: change the sheets on the bed.

FOOD:

A cloud of vanilla pudding.

Tip of the Day:

Patients with a brain illness often have sleeping problems.

Limit daytime napping. Keep the patient busy during the daytime hours. Keep the house dark and quiet around bedtime. Don't force the issue—that could make sleep a stressful experience. New studies even indicate that the patient should be allowed to sleep when they want to, if possible.

Quote of the Day:

"A good laugh and a long sleep are the best cures in the doctor's book."

~ Irish Proverb

Patient notes for today:

Physical or mental changes: _____

_____

_____

_____

Memory changes: _____

_____

_____

_____

Behavioral changes and triggers: _____

_____

_____

_____

Successes: _____

_____

_____

Challenges: _____

_____

_____

Seizure notes: _____

_____

_____

Medication or doctor notes: _____

_____

_____

_____

Pain level: _____

Energy level: _____

Rest or sleep issues: _____

Speech or word patterns: _____

Overall mood displayed by the patient:

_____
_____
_____
_____

Emotional expressions by the patient:

_____
_____
_____
_____

Caregiver feelings:

Today's feeling is (circle one) a **blessing** or a released **burden**:

_____
_____
_____
_____
_____
_____
_____
_____
_____
_____
_____
_____
_____
_____

Other notes:

To do list:

FLOWERS

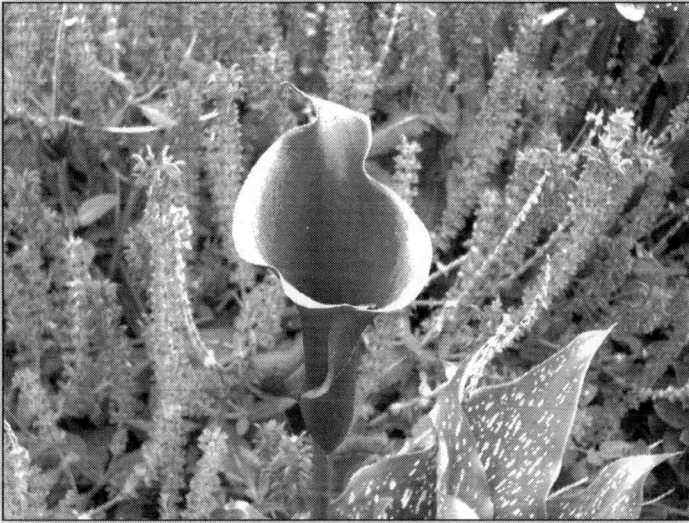

A living testimony to Mother Nature's beauty; I wish you could see the color of this beautiful, burgundy calla lily. Delicate and strikingly pure, you just want to stop and stare in awe.

~Photo by Joni Aldrich

The most significant calla lily meaning is magnificence and beauty. The calla lily name finds its origin from a Greek word for beauty. Roman legend has it that when Venus rose from the sea-foam, she saw a lily and became filled with jealous envy at the beauty of it. Seeing it as a rival to her own beauty, she caused a huge and monstrous pistil to spring from the lily's center. She obviously didn't succeed in destroying the beauty of this perfect flower.

Date: _____

SONGS:

Daisy Bell (composed by Harry Dacre—inspired by Daisy Greville, Countess of Warwick, a British socialite and mistress of King Edward VII)

Build Me Up Buttercup (written by Mike D'Abo and Tony Macaulay)

Roses are Red (lyrics by Al Byron)

ACTIVITIES:
- Visit a florist; take time to smell the roses.
- Paint beautiful flowers in an array of colors.
- Plant some herb or flower seeds, and watch the babies sprout.
- Make a silk flower arrangement.

FOOD:
Cauliflower

Tip of the Day:

Counseling is not for the weak—it's for the strong.

There is a stigma related to admitting that you need some extra help to get through some mental and emotional issues. In times when life gets tough, finding people to help you sort out your feelings and give you a better perspective is smart. Join a local support group. Share your feelings with family and friends.

Quote of the Day:

"Never apologize for showing feeling. When you do so you apologize for truth."

~ Benjamin Disraeli

Patient notes for today:

Physical or mental changes: _____

_____

_____

_____

Memory changes: _____

_____

_____

_____

Behavioral changes and triggers: _____

_____

_____

_____

Successes: _____

_____

_____

Challenges: _____

_____

_____

Seizure notes: _____

_____

_____

Medication or doctor notes: _____

_____

_____

_____

Pain level: _____

Energy level: _____

Rest or sleep issues: _____

Speech or word patterns: _____

Overall mood displayed by the patient:

_____
_____
_____
_____

Emotional expressions by the patient:

_____
_____
_____
_____

Caregiver feelings:

Today's feeling is (circle one) a **blessing** or a released **burden:**

_____
_____
_____
_____
_____
_____
_____
_____
_____
_____
_____
_____
_____
_____
_____

Other notes:

To do list:

Date: _____

Theme of the Day:
Love is in the Air

SONGS:

She Loves You (lyrics by John Lennon and Paul McCartney)

Love is a Many-Splendored Thing (lyrics by Paul Francis Webster)

Love Potion No. 9 (written by Jerry Leiber and Mike Stoller)

ACTIVITIES:
- Read love poetry. Try writing your own.
- Make a collage of pictures of those that you love.
- Make greeting cards; kits are available at your local craft store.

FOOD:
Chocolate

Tip of the Day:
Say this emphatically and often: "I love you unconditionally."

Words of comfort and affection will help to reassure and soothe the care receiver. Push aside other less important things to express your feelings of affection. Replace negative emotions with a simple declaration of love.

Quote of the Day:
"They do not love that do not show their love. The course of true love never did run smooth."

~ William Shakespeare

Patient notes for today:

Physical or mental changes: _____

_____

_____

_____

Memory changes: _____

_____

_____

_____

Behavioral changes and triggers: _____

_____

_____

_____

Successes: _____

_____

_____

Challenges: _____

_____

_____

Seizure notes: _____

_____

_____

Medication or doctor notes:_____

_____

_____

_____

Pain level: _____

Energy level: _____

Rest or sleep issues: _____

Speech or word patterns:_____

Overall mood displayed by the patient:

_____

_____

_____

_____

Emotional expressions by the patient:

_____

_____

_____

_____

Caregiver feelings:

Today's feeling is (circle one) a blessing or a released burden:

_____

_____

_____

_____

_____

_____

_____

_____

_____

_____

_____

_____

_____

_____

_____

_____

Other notes:

_____
_____
_____
_____
_____
_____
_____
_____
_____
_____
_____
_____

To do list:

_____
_____
_____
_____
_____
_____
_____
_____
_____
_____
_____
_____
_____
_____

Date: _____

SONGS:

Give My Regards to Broadway (written by George M. Cohan)

On Broadway (lyrics by Jerry Leiber and Mike Stoller)

Lullaby of Broadway (lyrics by Al Dubin)

ACTIVITIES:

- Watch some happy Broadway musicals (*not* Les Miserables).
- Talk about your favorite Broadway plays.
- Stage your own simple play. Have fun with it.

FOOD:

Hot dogs

Tip of the Day:

It's a "we" thing—who's in this with you for support?

A support group composed of family and friends is absolutely critical. Keeping all facets of life within balance can be an overwhelming effort. Even simple things like helping around the house and spending time with the patient are invaluable. Assistance may come in many different forms and functions—asking for the help that you need is the most direct approach.

Quote of the Day:

"Asking for help does not mean we are weak or incompetent. It usually indicates an advanced level of honesty and intelligence."

~ Anne Wilson Schaef

Patient notes for today:

Physical or mental changes: _____

_____

_____

_____

Memory changes: _____

_____

_____

_____

Behavioral changes and triggers: _____

_____

_____

_____

Successes: _____

_____

_____

Challenges: _____

_____

_____

Seizure notes: _____

_____

_____

Medication or doctor notes: _____

_____

_____

_____

Pain level: _____

Energy level: _____

Rest or sleep issues: _____

Speech or word patterns: _____

Overall mood displayed by the patient:

_____

_____

_____

_____

Emotional expressions by the patient:

_____

_____

_____

_____

Caregiver feelings:

Today's feeling is (circle one) a **blessing** or a released **burden**:

_____

_____

_____

_____

_____

_____

_____

_____

_____

_____

_____

_____

_____

_____

_____

_____

_____

Other notes:

To do list:

FLY ME TO THE MOON

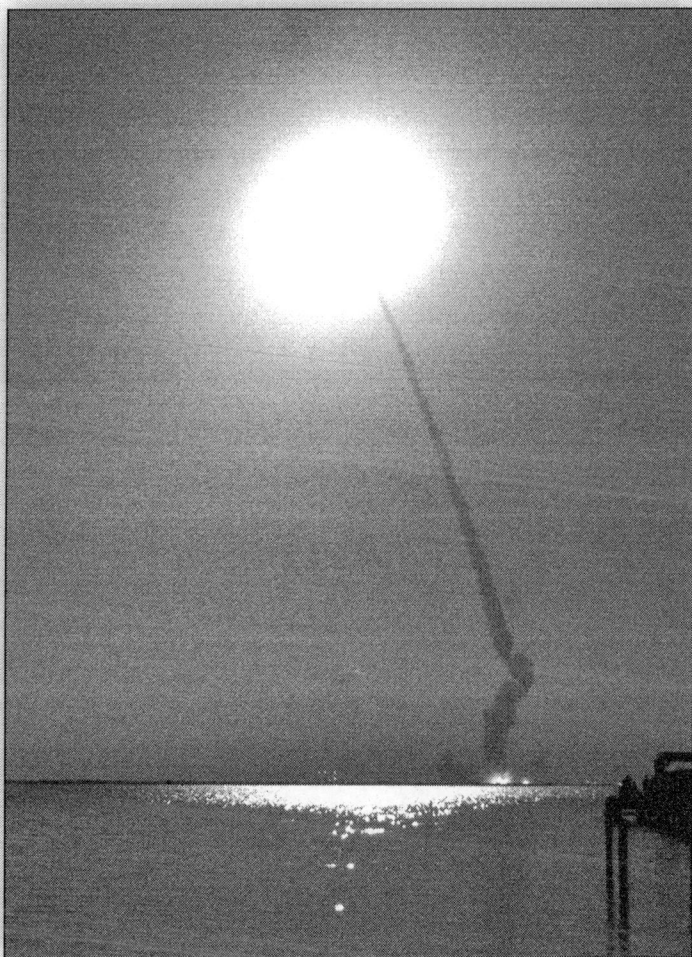

This picture was taken during one of the final space shuttle launches of 2010—and perhaps forever! It's an awesome spectacle to see the power and beauty of a rocket or shuttle launch, especially at night.

~*Photo by Joni Aldrich*

News from July 20th, 1969:

Anyone who was alive that day will tell you they remember the excitement. For thousands of years, mankind had looked to the heavens and dreamed of walking on the moon. As part of the Apollo 11 mission, dream became reality. At 4:18 p.m., the Eagle landed on the moon's surface in the Sea of Tranquility. Neil Armstrong then turned on the cameras that would transmit images from the moon to billions of people who sat glued to their televisions. He climbed down a ladder, and became the first person to set foot on the moon at 10:56 p.m. Armstrong's first words were: "That's one small step for man, one giant leap for mankind." This amazing accomplishment gave people around the world hope of future space exploration.

Date: _____

Fly Me to the Moon

SONGS:

Fly Me to the Moon (written by Bart Howard)

Blue Moon (lyrics by Lorenz Hart)

Moon River (lyrics by Johnny Mercer)

ACTIVITIES:

- Look at a book about the planets and star formations.
- Draw the planets and stars.
- Visit a planetarium, or look through a telescope at the stars.

FOOD:

Swiss cheese

Tip of the Day:

The needs and feelings of the caregiver are important, too!

If you don't get enough rest and try to do all of the work yourself, you risk harm to the care receiver and your own personal health. When faced with the task of caregiving, many people run their health into the ground. That is a lose-lose situation.

Quote of the Day:

"One person caring about another represents life's greatest value."

~ Jim Rohn

Patient notes for today:

Physical or mental changes: _____

_____

_____

_____

Memory changes: _____

_____

_____

_____

Behavioral changes and triggers: _____

_____

_____

_____

Successes: _____

_____

_____

Challenges: _____

_____

_____

Seizure notes: _____

_____

_____

Medication or doctor notes:_____

_____

_____

_____

Pain level: _____

Energy level: _____

Rest or sleep issues: _____

Speech or word patterns:_____

Overall mood displayed by the patient:

_____

_____

_____

_____

Emotional expressions by the patient:

_____

_____

_____

_____

Caregiver feelings:

Today's feeling is (circle one) a **blessing** or a released **burden**:

_____

_____

_____

_____

_____

_____

_____

_____

_____

_____

_____

_____

_____

_____

Other notes:

To do list:

Date: _____

Elvis is Still King

SONGS:

Love Me Tender (based on *Aura Lee*, words by W.W. Fosdick)

Hound Dog (lyrics by Jerry Leiber and Mike Stoller)

Blue Suede Shoes (written and first recorded by Carl Perkins)

ACTIVITIES:
- Watch some Elvis movies.
- Create an Elvis collage.
- Practice some smooth Elvis dance moves (just don't blow out your knees)!

FOOD:

Elvis Presley's favorite sandwich was peanut butter, banana and bacon. You might want to have Memphis barbecue instead.

Tip of the Day:

Regroup rather than repeat.

If the listener doesn't receive the message the first time, they're not likely to understand it exactly the same way the second time. Try a slightly different tactic, and you may get better results.

Quote of the Day:

"What is the use of running, if you are not on the right road?"

~German proverb

Patient notes for today:

Physical or mental changes: _____

_____

_____

_____

Memory changes: _____

_____

_____

_____

Behavioral changes and triggers: _____

_____

_____

_____

Successes: _____

_____

_____

Challenges: _____

_____

_____

Seizure notes: _____

_____

_____

Medication or doctor notes:_____

_____

_____

_____

Pain level: _____

Energy level: _____

Rest or sleep issues: _____

Speech or word patterns:_____

Overall mood displayed by the patient:

_____

_____

_____

_____

Emotional expressions by the patient:

_____

_____

_____

_____

Caregiver feelings:

Today's feeling is (circle one) a **blessing** or a released **burden:**

_____

_____

_____

_____

_____

_____

_____

_____

_____

_____

_____

_____

_____

_____

_____

_____

Other notes:

To do list:

Date: _____

Oldies Goldies ('50s and '60s)

SONGS:

Unchained Melody (lyrics by Hy Zaret)

Great Balls of Fire (written by Otis Blackwell and Jack Hammer)

All I Have to Do Is Dream (written by Boudleaux Bryant)

ACTIVITIES:

- Talk about your favorite memories of the '50s and '60s.
- Name as many performers from that era as you can.
- Create your own diner or drive-in, or visit one in your area.
- Have a karaoke day!

FOOD:

Burger and fries (at the drive-in)

Tip of the Day:

Music has the power to bring back memories and reduce stress.

Music has a unique link to our emotions. As music absorbs our attention, it acts as a distraction away from more serious concerns. The rhythm makes us want to tap our feet and clap our hands.

Quote of the Day:

**"My goal in life is to give to the world what I was lucky to receive...
the ecstasy of divine union through my music and my dance."**

~ Mick Jagger

Patient notes for today:

Physical or mental changes: _____

_____

_____

_____

Memory changes: _____

_____

_____

_____

Behavioral changes and triggers: _____

_____

_____

_____

Successes: _____

_____

_____

Challenges: _____

_____

_____

Seizure notes: _____

_____

_____

Medication or doctor notes: _____

_____

_____

_____

Pain level: _____

Energy level: _____

Rest or sleep issues: _____

Speech or word patterns: _____

Overall mood displayed by the patient:

_____
_____
_____
_____

Emotional expressions by the patient:

_____
_____
_____
_____

Caregiver feelings:

Today's feeling is (circle one) a **blessing** or a released **burden**:

_____
_____
_____
_____
_____
_____
_____
_____
_____
_____
_____
_____
_____
_____
_____
_____

Other notes:

To do list:

DISNEY MAGIC

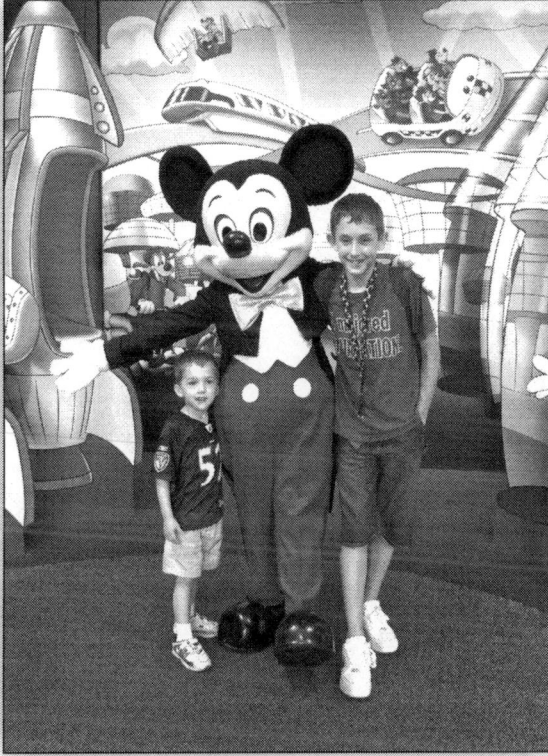

Mickey Mouse is handsome, but the two good-looking young men in this picture get the prize. They are my very own grandchildren! Dawson is on the left, and Dallas is on the right.

~Photo by Joni Aldrich

> Grandparents and grandchildren;
> Together they create a chain of love
> Linking the past with the future.
> The chain may lengthen,
> But it will never part.

(Unknown Author)

Date: _____

Disney Magic

SONGS:

When You Wish Upon A Star (lyrics by Ned Washington)

The Mickey Mouse Club March (written by host Jimmie Dodd)

Zip-a-Dee-Doo-Dah (lyrics by Ray Gilbert)

ACTIVITIES:

- Watch Disney movies or cartoons. Stay away from ones with mean villains like Cruella de Vil. Stick with Mickey or Goofy.
- Talk about your favorite Disney characters.
- Read the history of Walt Disney.

FOOD:

Make a Mickey Mouse head with two small and one large chocolate chip cookies.

Tip of the Day:

Create moments of success and joy for your care receiver.

Try to enrich your care receiver's life by creating moments of success and joy, sidestepping moments of failure, and praising their efforts with gusto. After all, aren't these the basic needs that we all want fulfilled?

Quote of the Day:

"Joy is a net of love by which you can catch souls."

~Mother Teresa

Patient notes for today:

Physical or mental changes: _____

_____

_____

_____

Memory changes: _____

_____

_____

_____

Behavioral changes and triggers: _____

_____

_____

_____

Successes: _____

_____

_____

Challenges: _____

_____

_____

Seizure notes: _____

_____

_____

Medication or doctor notes: _____

_____

_____

_____

Pain level: _____

Energy level: _____

Rest or sleep issues: _____

Speech or word patterns: _____

Overall mood displayed by the patient:

_____

_____

_____

_____

Emotional expressions by the patient:

_____

_____

_____

_____

Caregiver feelings:

Today's feeling is (circle one) a **blessing** or a released **burden**:

_____

_____

_____

_____

_____

_____

_____

_____

_____

_____

_____

_____

_____

_____

_____

_____

_____

Other notes:

To do list:

Date: _____

Believing in Magic

SONGS:

Do You Believe in Magic (written by John Sebastian)

That Old Black Magic (lyrics by Johnny Mercer)

Puff, the Magic Dragon (based on a poem by Leonard Lipton)

ACTIVITIES:

- Get a magic kit, or make up some magic moves of your own.
- Make up your own card tricks.
- Sort cards, buttons, or poker chips.

FOOD:

Herbs: parsley, sage, rosemary, and thyme.

Tip of the Day:

Become proficient at the art of distraction.

Sometimes the subject may panic you, but it's important to keep a clear head. If the patient asks for the car keys, discuss why they want to have them. It may take the topic in a different direction. For example, if they say they need them to go to church, ask them why they like church. The conversation may go towards that topic—and away from driving.

Quote of the Day:

"The mind gets distracted in all sorts of ways. The heart is its own exclusive concern and diversion."

~Malcolm de Chazal

Patient notes for today:

Physical or mental changes: _____

_____

_____

_____

Memory changes: _____

_____

_____

_____

Behavioral changes and triggers: _____

_____

_____

_____

Successes: _____

_____

_____

Challenges: _____

_____

_____

Seizure notes: _____

_____

_____

Medication or doctor notes:_____

_____

_____

_____

Pain level: _____

Energy level: _____

Rest or sleep issues: _____

Speech or word patterns:_____

Overall mood displayed by the patient:

_____
_____
_____
_____

Emotional expressions by the patient:

_____
_____
_____
_____

Caregiver feelings:

Today's feeling is (circle one) a **blessing** or a released **burden**:

_____
_____
_____
_____
_____
_____
_____
_____
_____
_____
_____
_____
_____
_____
_____

Other notes:

_____
_____
_____
_____
_____
_____
_____
_____
_____
_____
_____
_____

To do list:

_____
_____
_____
_____
_____
_____
_____
_____
_____
_____
_____
_____
_____
_____

Date: _____

Celebration Time!

SONGS:

Celebration (written by Donna Johnson and Kool and the Gang)

For He's a Jolly Good Fellow (unknown, but very popular)

Auld Lang Syne (based on a Scots poem written by Robert Burns)

ACTIVITIES:
- Make up a reason to have a party!
- Discuss reasons that we celebrate.
- Give each other gold stars.

FOOD:
Cake

Tip of the Day:

Bad moods can be reflected in the patient.

Moods—good or bad—are infectious. If the caregiver projects a gloomy attitude, it can rub off on the patient. While it may be impossible to be cheery every day, scheduling things that are fun for both the caregiver and patient will help to boost the atmosphere away from gloom.

Quote of the Day:

**"The trick is to be grateful when your mood
is high, and graceful when it is low."**

~Richard Carlson

Patient notes for today:

Physical or mental changes: _____

_____

_____

_____

Memory changes: _____

_____

_____

_____

Behavioral changes and triggers: _____

_____

_____

_____

Successes: _____

_____

_____

Challenges: _____

_____

_____

Seizure notes: _____

_____

_____

Medication or doctor notes:_____

_____

_____

_____

Pain level: _____

Energy level: _____

Rest or sleep issues: _____

Speech or word patterns:_____

Overall mood displayed by the patient:

_____
_____
_____
_____

Emotional expressions by the patient:

_____
_____
_____
_____

Caregiver feelings:

Today's feeling is (circle one) a **blessing** or a released **burden**:

_____
_____
_____
_____
_____
_____
_____
_____
_____
_____
_____
_____
_____
_____

Other notes:

_____
_____
_____
_____
_____
_____
_____
_____
_____
_____
_____
_____

To do list:

_____
_____
_____
_____
_____
_____
_____
_____
_____
_____
_____
_____
_____

8263622R1

Made in the USA
Charleston, SC
24 May 2011